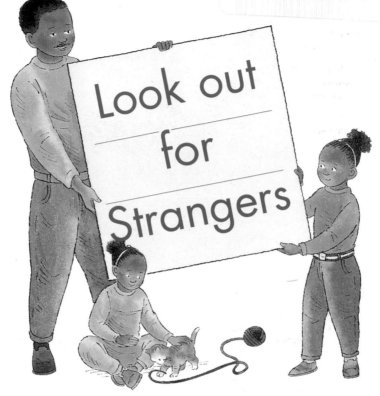

Look out
for
Strangers

Paul Humphrey and
Alex Ramsay

Illustrated by
Colin King

Evans

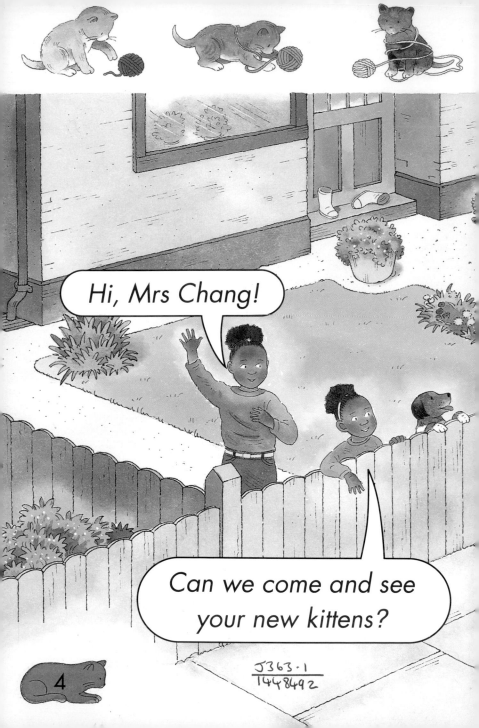

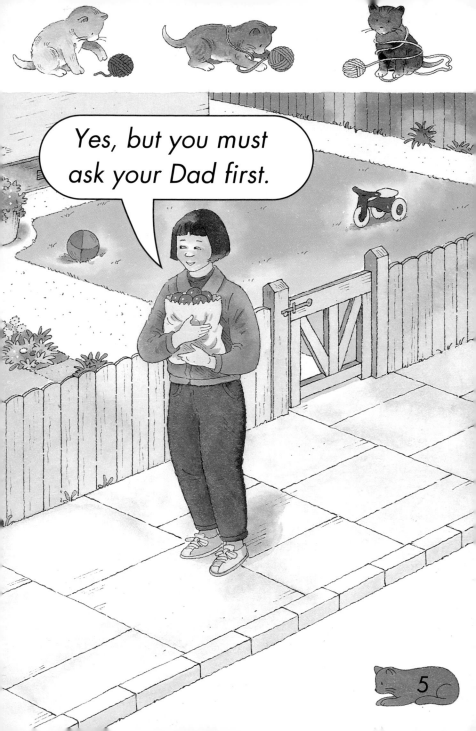

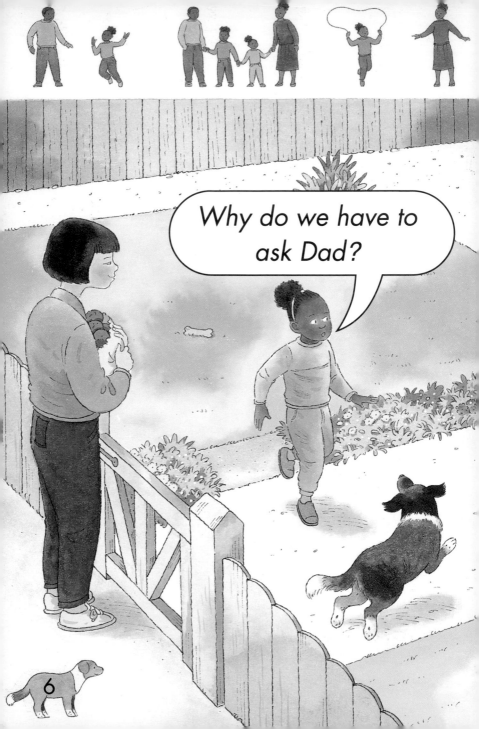

6

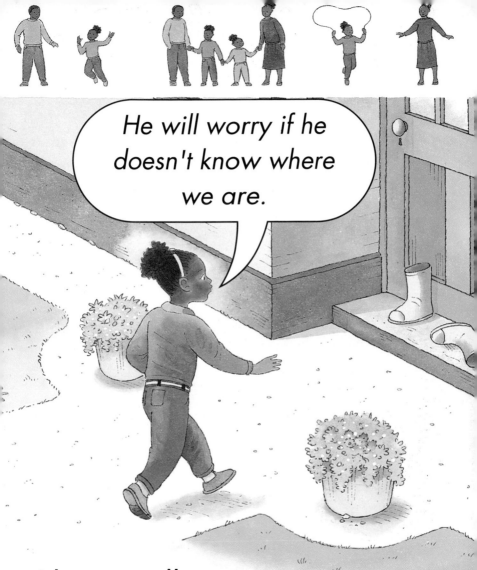

Always tell your parents
where you are going.

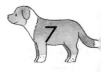

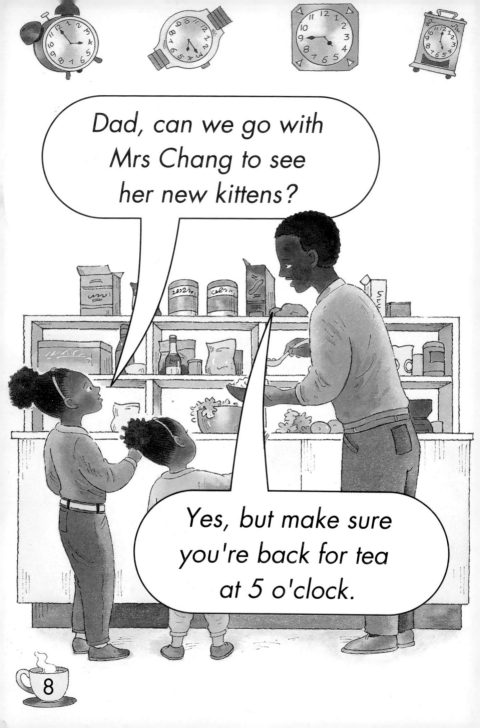

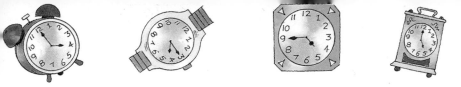

Mum or Dad must know what time you are coming home.

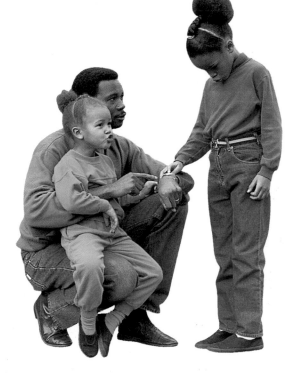

Then they can come and find you if they are worried.

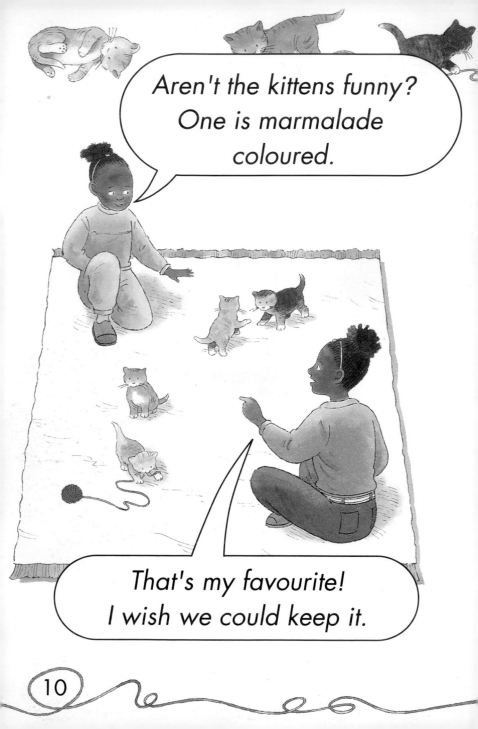

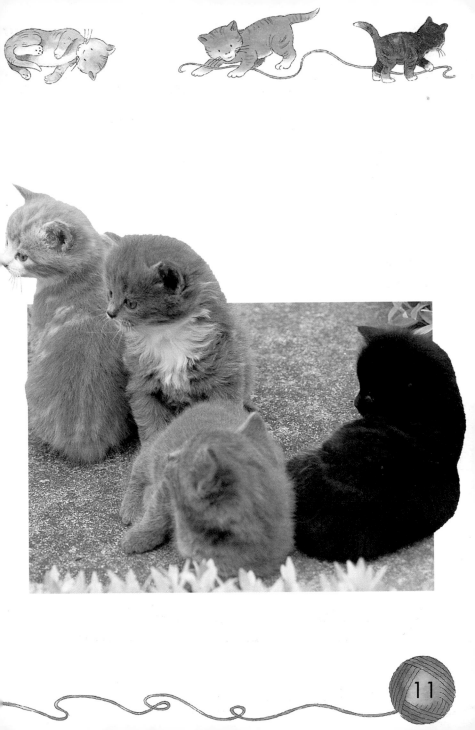

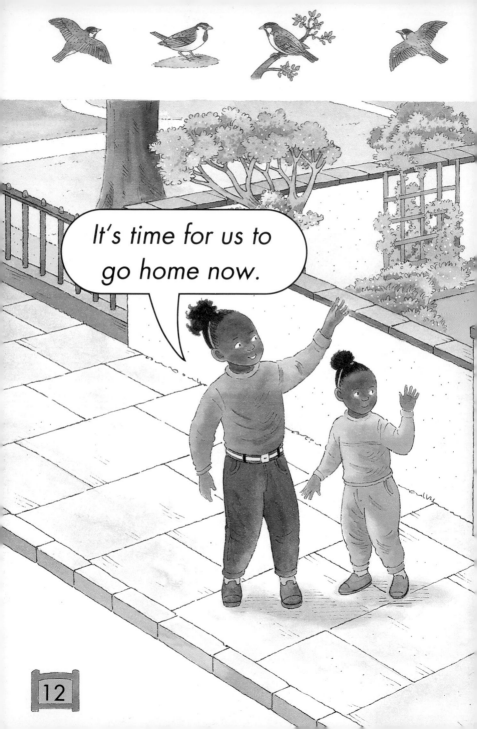

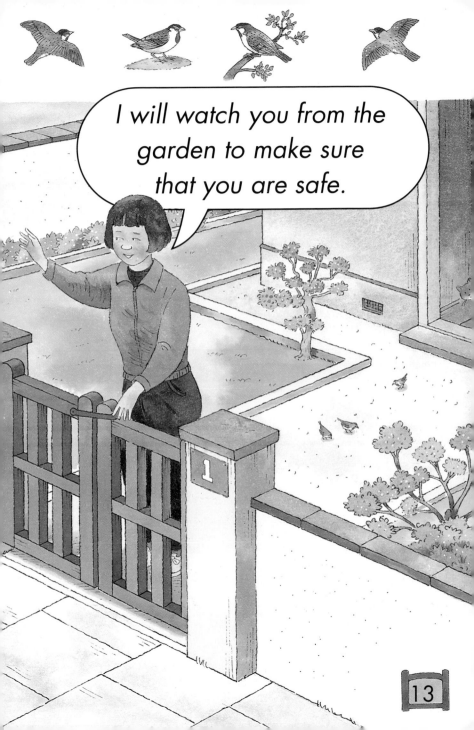

13

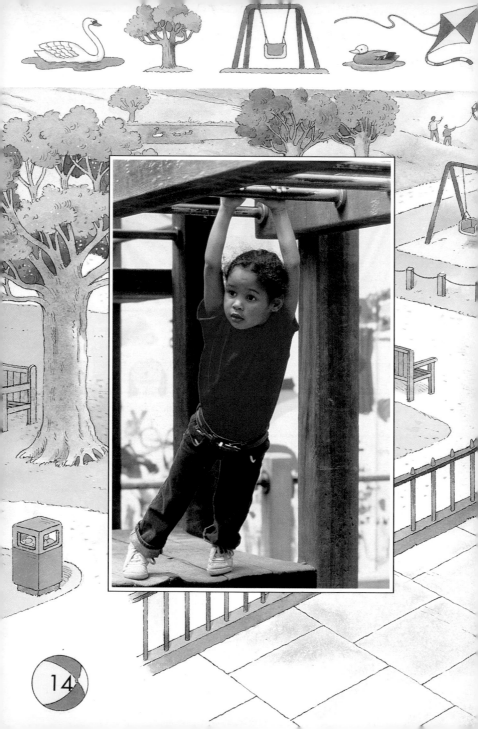

14

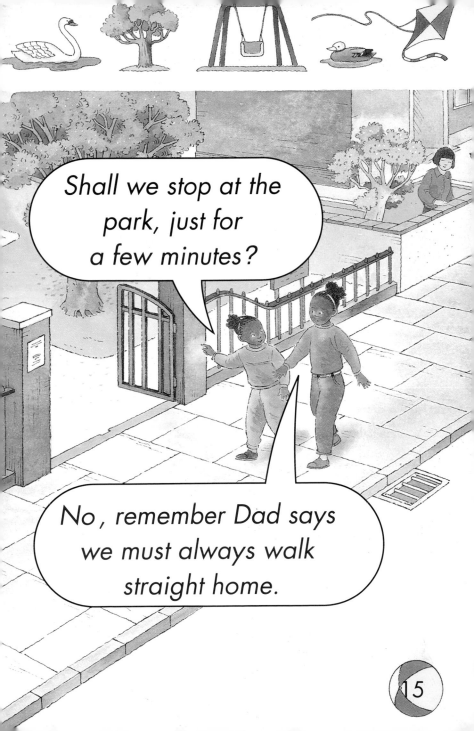

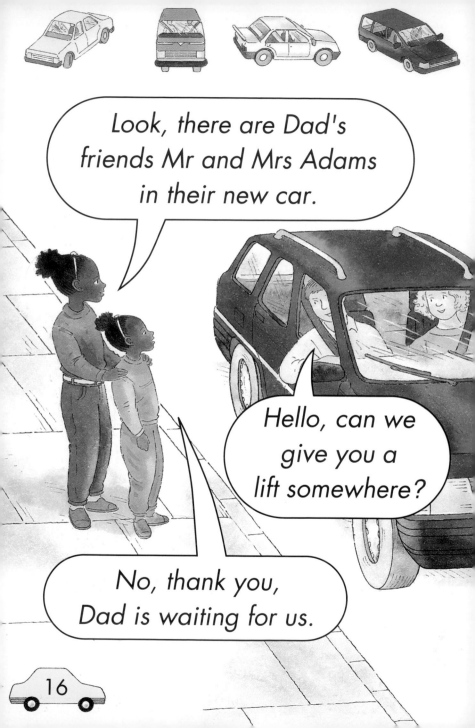

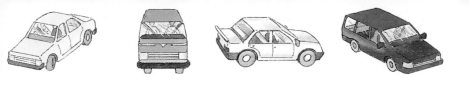

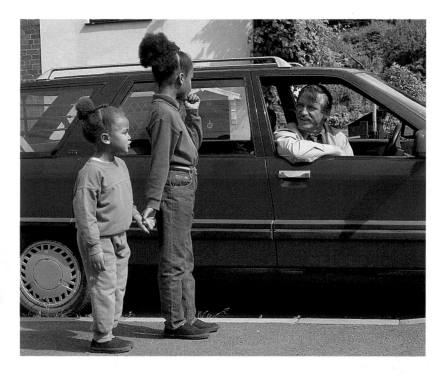

Never get in a car with someone, even if you know them, without asking Mum or Dad first.

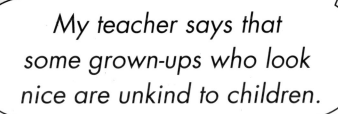

My teacher says that some grown-ups who look nice are unkind to children.

That's right. We should never go with anyone even if they say Mum or Dad told them to pick us up.

Remember, it's not rude to say no. Nice grown-ups will never mind you saying it.

19

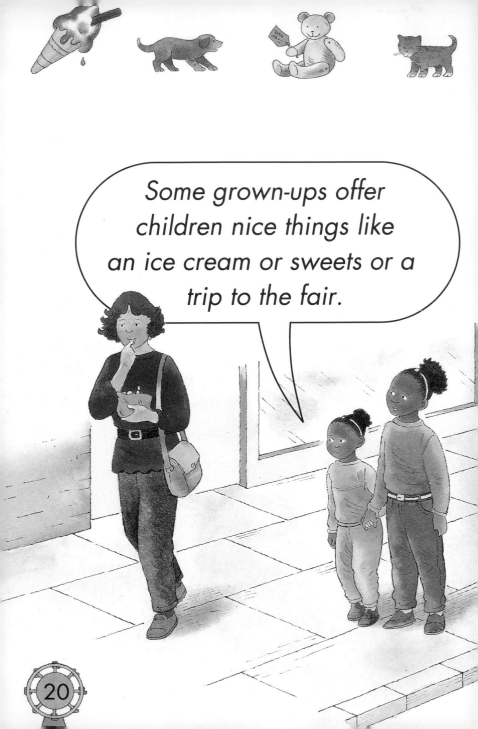

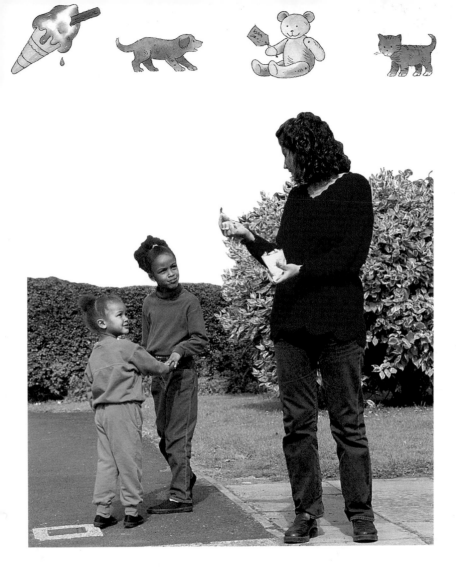

Always say no if a stranger offers you treats.

21

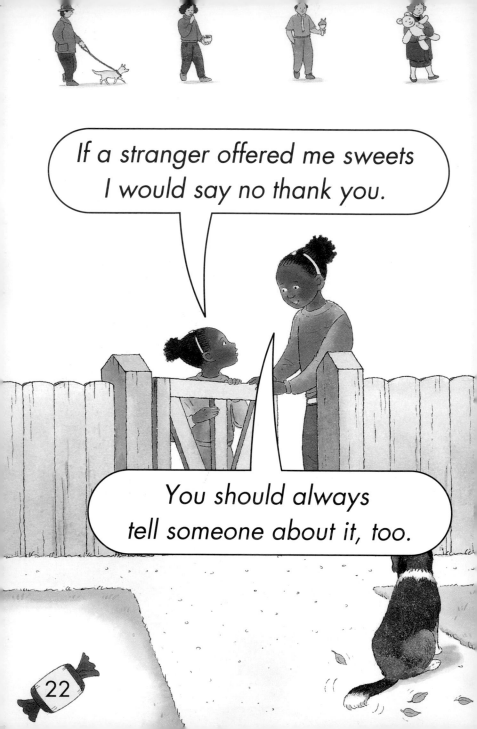

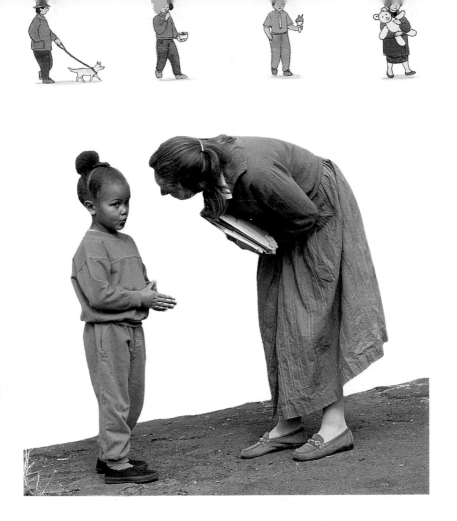

You can tell your teacher,
your parents or grandparents
or a police officer.

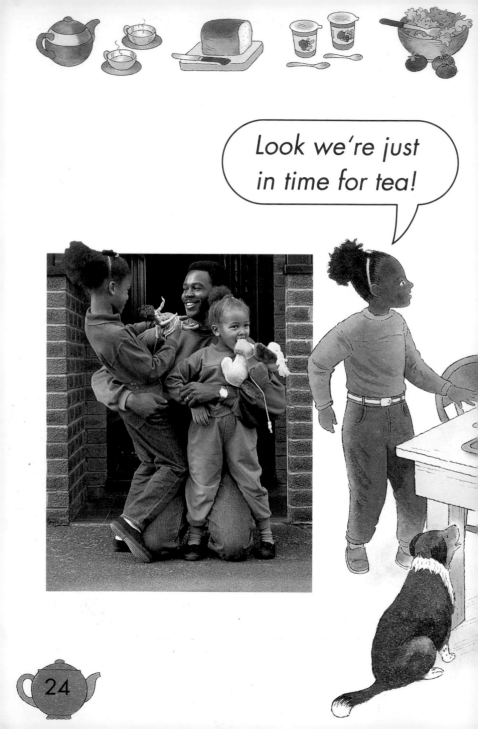

Look we're just in time for tea!

24

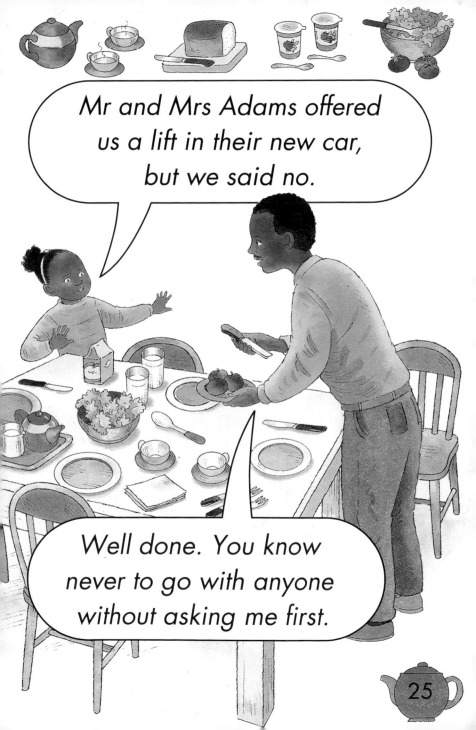

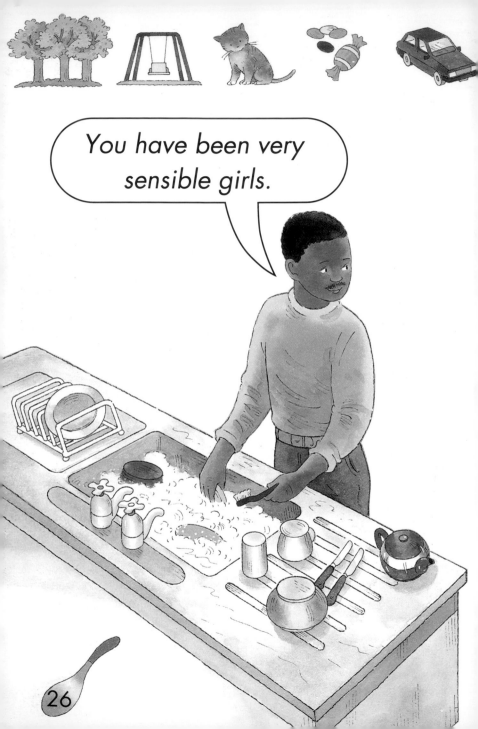

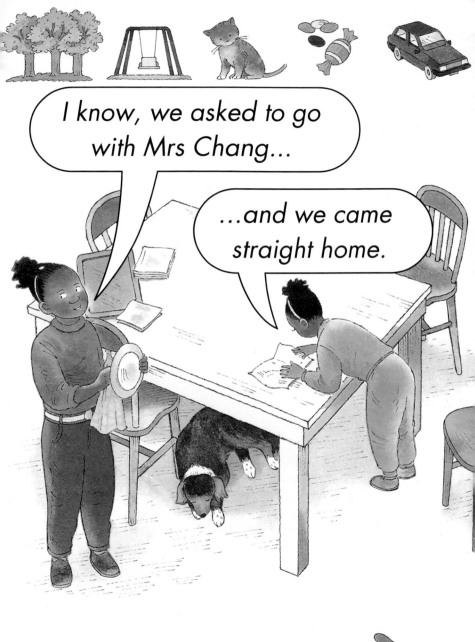

27

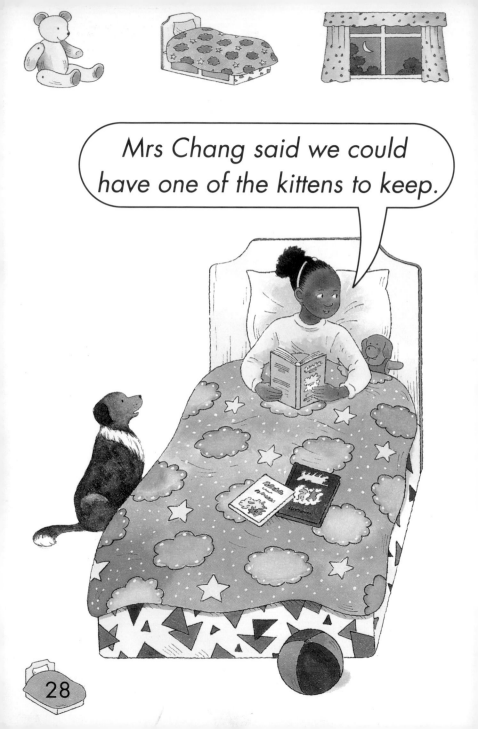

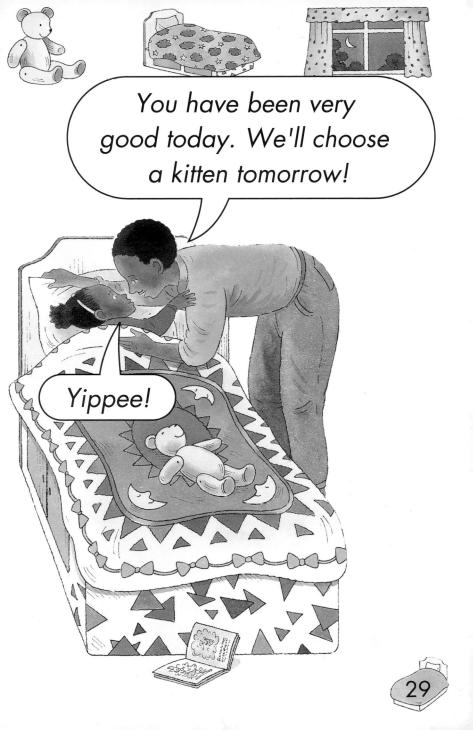

29

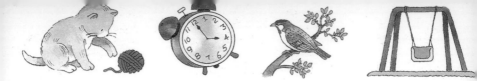

Some rules to remember:

1. Make sure your Mum or Dad knows where you are (see pages **6 - 8**).

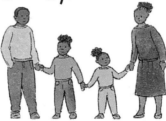

2. Make sure Mum or Dad knows when you are coming home (see pages **8 - 9**).

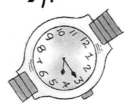

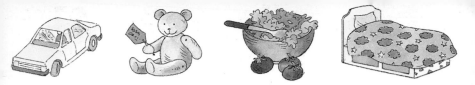

3. Never get in a car or go with someone without asking Mum or Dad first (see pages **16 - 19**).

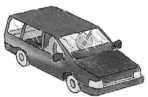

4. Never talk to strangers or take treats from them (see pages **20 - 23**).

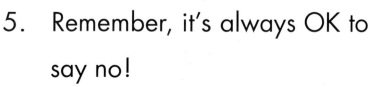

5. Remember, it's always OK to say no!